The Calcium Magnesium Magic Revealed

"Discover The Best Way To Use Calcium: Magnesium To Eliminate Illness"

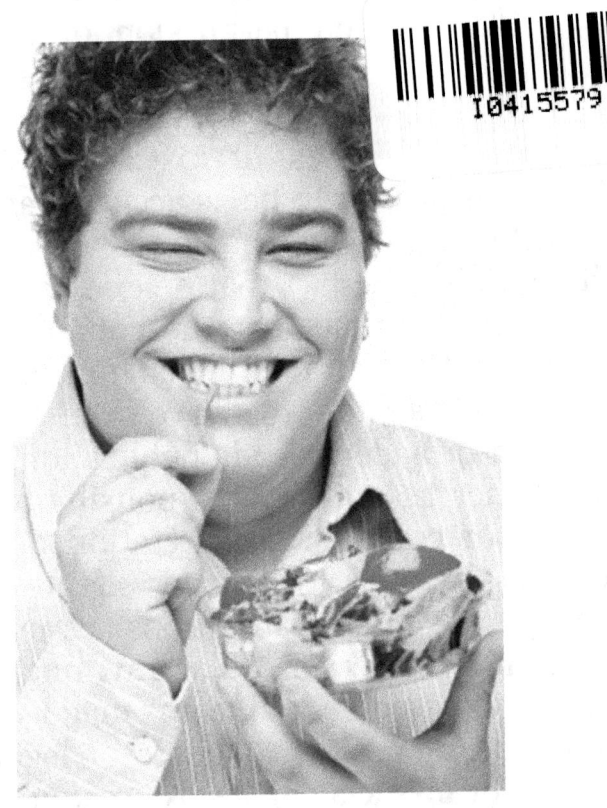

I0415579

Rudy S Silva, Natural Nutritionist

The Calcium Magnesium Magic Revealed, © 2013 by Rudy S Silva

ISBN-13: 978-1492929192
ISBN-10: 1492929190

Disclaimer and Terms of Use: The Author and Publisher has strived to be as accurate and complete as possible in the creation of this book, notwithstanding the fact that he does not warrant or represent at any time that the contents within are accurate due to the rapidly changing nature of the Internet. While all attempts have been made to verify information provided in this publication, the Author and Publisher assumes no responsibility for errors, omissions, or contrary interpretation of the subject matter herein. Any perceived slights of specific persons, peoples, or organizations are unintentional. In practical advice books, like anything else in life, there are no guarantees of income made. This book is not intended for use as a source of legal, business, accounting or financial advice. All readers are advised to seek services of competent professionals in legal, business, accounting, and finance field.

Your doctor or health provider should confirm any information given here. This information should not be taken as medical advice or treatment. This e-book is for information and educational purposes only. Consult with your doctor before using any of the remedies, recommendations, or information listed in this e-book.

First Printing, 2013, Printed in the United States of America

Table of Contents

Introduction: The Importance Of Calcium

Calcium occurs in the earth as limestone, calcium carbonate, as gypsum, or as apatite. It is always found combined with other elements. You will never find a pure calcium rock.

When these types of calcium compounds combine with water, they dissolve and form an alkaline solution. This is one of the reasons why you want to know as much about calcium, since it is one of the main elements that can make your body liquids alkaline.

One of the most important health programs you need to pursue is to move your body from an acid condition into an alkaline condition, and calcium helps you do this.

When your body is maintained consistently in an acid condition, calcium is also constantly removed from your bones, which results in porous bones, or from tissue or organs causing degradation of those areas.

Calcium is the most abundant of the minerals in your body, and it makes up 1.6% of your body weight or represents 40% of all the minerals in your body. But, 99% of the calcium you have is located in your bones. The other 1% is distributed throughout your body, and it's involved in numerous structural and biochemical processes throughout your body.

Bone Loss

Bone loss starts around middle age. For women, it increases during menopause. For men, bone loss is slow but steady starting from around 30. In bone loss, there are normally no symptoms. But here are a few that stand out:
Bone deformity or rickets
Muscle and leg cramps
Insomnia
Growth retardation

Unfortunately, around 40% of women who live over 75 years will experience bone loss fractures. Here are some reasons for low bone mass at any age.

Diet that lacks the daily use of fruits and vegetables
Slender body or low weight
Premature menopause
Anorexia nervosa
Extreme athletic training
Lack of exercise or a sedentary lifestyle
Excess eating or using various types of meat or protein, phosphorus, sodium, caffeine, wheat bran, and alcohol
Smoking
Excess use of sodas
Use of corticosteroid medications
Prolong bed rest or confined to a wheel chair

It has been found that if you lack a small drop in the required level of calcium in your body, this deficiency will activate aging and many degenerative diseases. Even though calcium is a large atom, it chemically moves 10,000 times faster and is 10,000 times stronger than magnesium.

This gives calcium the ability to bind quickly and strongly with important biological molecules, which sustain life. This chemical flexibility gives calcium the honor of being called "the King of the Bioelements."

In this kindle e-book, you will discover why it has this name. Despite there is more calcium in the body than any other mineral, except for oxygen, calcium is not more important than the other minerals, since all work together and are needed in your body for maintaining life.

What we can say about calcium is that it is involved in more biochemical activities in your body than any other mineral, so that it is important to supply your body with a good amount of calcium. Your body will eliminate the excess calcium from your body as its natural behavior, even when it is in a super saturated form in your body liquids.

But, when there is a deficiency of other minerals in your body that must balance with calcium, like sodium, excess calcium can react un-naturally, causing calcium crystalline deposits, which lead to pain and disease.

When your body lacks calcium and has unhealthy or porous bones, calcium will deposit calcium crystalline stones in various places in your body as it tries to build up weak bones. A misconception is that if you have calcium deposits in the joints or tissue giving you pain, that you have too much calcium.

The truth is you do not have enough calcium, so the body tries to compensate for this by a calcium deposit to build your bones back up.

Calcium is found in your blood, bone structure, tissue, muscles, lymph liquid, and in every body cell in your body. It is found in the lymph liquid outside and inside your cells. In the so-called **Sodium – Potassium Pump** the mineral sodium moves out of the cell and moves potassium into the cell. When the inside of the cell has mostly potassium, the electric charge inside the cell is less than the charge outside of the cell where sodium dominates. This condition attracts calcium to carry food nutrients into the cell and to perform in the cells various biochemical and bioelectrical reactions.

Calcium ions also play a major role in nerve stimulations and transmissions, muscle contractions and movements, and organ hormone secretions and many other biological functions. It is involved with your body's enzymes to produce energy.

Calcium ions concentrations are the most regulated mineral in your blood plasma. Its ionic form is Ca^{++} and in this form its most important function is in nerve function. For nerve function, calcium keeps your nerves receptive to sodium ions, which help to transmit brain impulses and information to various parts of the body, which regulate your body's activities.

In those cultures where drinking water had a high content of calcium, it was found that people's life span was 10 years or more than in western countries.

Kidneys

Your kidneys act as filters for your blood and they remove those nutrients or chemicals that your body no longer needs from your blood and this includes calcium. Excess calcium is routed to your bladder where it is expelled in your urine. If calcium is still needed, your kidneys will pass it into your blood to be reused by your body.

Most minerals and vitamins combine and react with calcium to produce the various body structures and chemicals that make up your body.

It was thought at one time that if you produced kidney stones that you needed to take less calcium. If you tend to form kidney stones, you will have increased calcium in your urine, but this is caused by your body pulling calcium out of your bones.

Because eating excess meat causes your body to excrete calcium it is recommended, for kidney stones, to eat less meat, increase the use of fruits and vegetables, and supplement with calcium citrate, magnesium, vitamin B6 and vitamin C.

You can take calcium citrate on an empty stomach. Most other supplements, you should take with meals.

Calcium Toxicity

Usually, there is no calcium toxicity, even when you take a large dose. There is some concern that people with a tendency toward kidney stones should avoid excess calcium, but these concerns have not been proven. Kidney stones are more related to dieting and those people who favor an acid diet tend to form kidney stones. In an acid diet, calcium is active and depleted as it is used up neutralizing body acids.

Chapter 1: The Magic Of Calcium In Your Body

Here is a list of some of the important biochemical and bioelectrical functions of calcium in the body:

Absorption of calcium
Activity in cell function
Maintaining an alkaline body
Contributing to Saliva alkaline body test
Needed Calcium foods

Adsorption of Calcium

Calcium is one of more difficult minerals to digest and to absorb through your intestinal walls. Various phosphates and other compounds (Phosphates are derived from phosphoric acid and when they combine with oxygen they become an organic phosphates, which have important biochemical activities in your body) found in red meat and sodas react with calcium to form a calcium phosphate precipitate. This prevents calcium from being absorbed and calcium is then excreted from your body.

However, when calcium comes in contact with the food substance of milk and various fruits and vegetables, it forms compounds that are easily absorbed.

For calcium to be absorbed into your body, it needs to have adequate vitamin D. Without Vitamin D, calcium cannot be absorbed into your blood stream. Vitamin D can be obtained from the sun and is critical in the amount of calcium absorption that occurs in your small intestine. This is why you need to get at least 20 minutes of sun every day. In some parts of the world, less time is needed and in other parts more time is needed.

You can also get vitamin D from supplements. Some foods have it, but in very small quantities. When the sun's UV light hits your skin, fatty acids in your skin create vitamin D and **Inositol triphosphate, INSP-3**. This vitamin D finds its way into your intestinal wall where it assists calcium to move through it and into your blood stream.

Inositol triphosphate finds its way into every body cell. Its function is to release calcium from storage from within your cells, when inadequate calcium is not provided by your diet and supplements, or when insufficient vitamin D causes less calcium to be absorbed in the intestinal wall.

Inositol is obtained from foods such as fruits, vegetables, grains, and from liver, kidney and heart.

When there is insufficient calcium in the cell walls, because it got used up, the parathyroid hormone stimulated by deficiency of vitamin D activates the extraction of calcium from your bones. Once the bones become weaken, your body starts extracting calcium from proteins that regulate your cell functions. This results in a variety of aliment and disease symptoms.

Once in your blood stream, calcium is deposited in bones with the help of the hormone, calcitonin, released by parathyroid gland. Also, both Calcitonin and Inositol triphosphate regulate the storage and removal of calcium with in the cells.

The parathyroid gland is regulated by the pituitary gland, which is right behind the eyes. When you wear sunglasses, this blocks the full-spectrum UV light that is needed to regulate the pituitary gland, so that it can produce the hormones needed to regulate calcium in your cells.

Without adequate amounts of vitamin D, calcium will not be absorbed in proper amounts into your body and will just pass right through, excreted from your body.

Parathyroid – How it regulates calcium

The parathyroid is actively involved in maintaining your calcium blood levels. These levels are maintained to a very strict range. When your blood calcium levels drop, the parathyroid releases a hormone that directs the release of calcium from your bones and into your blood stream. And at the same time, it tells your kidneys not to excrete calcium into your urine.

Now, when you have excess calcium in your blood, the amount of the parathyroid hormone secreted is decreased. This causes the kidneys to expel more calcium into your urine. As all of this is happening, the parathyroid also releases a hormone called Calcitonin, which reduces the amount of calcium that is pull out of your bones.

Activity in cell function

Calcium is active in the process involving the Sodium-Potassium Pump in that it uses this pump to enter and exit from a cell. When it enters the cell, it brings in food nutrients to feed the cells. Once it releases these nutrients, it becomes a free ion. As these calcium ions build up in the cell, the voltage across the cell membrane will again reaches 70 millivolts. This sets the stage for nutrients and toxins in the cell to be pushed out of the cell and for other nutrients to enter the cell.

Maintaining an alkaline body

The fluid outside the cells is called extracellular fluid. This fluid is maintained at a pH of 7.4 by a calcium compound called calcium mono orthophosphate. This fluid is capable of neutralizing acids that come out of the cells or arrive there from food that you have eaten. Sodium is also in the extracellular fluid and can neutralize acids, but it is needed in large quantities to maintain the Sodium-Potassium Pump cell activity. Wherever calcium is in the tissue, joints, blood, liquid or organs, it will neutralize acids. This process reduces damage to your tissues and elevates your body pH, making it more alkaline.

When you don't have enough calcium in your body, the cells will not have enough calcium to neutralize body acids and this will cause cell deterioration and will lead to various diseases. Keeping your body liquid alkaline or with a pH above 6.8 to 7.5 is what you should be working towards with any health program that you are working with. This can be done by using the right alkaline diet.

An alkaline diet helps you balance the level of acid and alkaline in all parts of your body. When you eat more acid foods, such as meat, butter, fats, carbohydrates, then your body needs to use up its alkaline stores to neutralize this acid, to prevent damage to your body's cells and tissue.

When you eat more alkaline foods than you need, you run the risk of not getting enough protein or carbohydrate and your pH can move above 7. 5 or 8.0, which can also lead to disease. You need a balance of certain foods to get your body pH in the range of 7.0.

The saliva alkaline body test

In other kindle e-books, the saliva test has been discussed so that you can check its pH. This test is a strong indicator of whether your calcium ion level is sufficient. Here is a review.

When your Saliva pH is 7.0 to 7.5, it is considered alkaline and normal. When this is the case, your urine will be slightly acidic. When you lack ionic calcium, your pH will be 4.6 to 6.4, and your urine will be tend to be acidic.

Now here is important information. If you have physical ailments, your pH will be from 6.0 to 6.5. In this case, you should take around 2000 mg of calcium rather than 1000 mg. If your pH is below 6.0, mostly likely, you will have various disease symptoms. And, you should be taking around 3000 mg of calcium. Once you bring up your salivary pH, you can lower your calcium intake.

If your saliva tests show your pH to be below 6.0, then by taking more calcium supplements and by eating more fruits and vegetable during the day and especially in the evening, you can change your pH to 6.5 to 7.5.

Keep in mind that the saliva test may not always be accurate, since the saliva pH can be influenced by food recently eaten. To get the most accurate reading, take the saliva test only after 2 hours of eating your last meal or snack. Also, bring saliva into your mouth 3 times and swallow, before taking the test. Take the test 3 times on 3 different days to make sure your readings are consistent.

In my kindle e-book called "Secret Diet and Nutrition

Tips 1: Alkaline Body" I show you how you can change your body from 6.0 pH to 7.0 pH.   In addition, in this e-book I show you how to do the saliva test properly so that you can get a good reading.

Simply changing your diet, taking vitamins, and mineral supplements when you eat, you can change your body's pH to the 7.0 to 7.5 level. When you do this, you will see a change in any physical aliment and disease that you might have.   It will not occur instantly. You will need to keep this pH level for a few months.

Chapter 2: Illnesses Caused by Lack of Calcium

Calcium plays a major role in blood, cells, liver, kidney, and heart health. Calcium maintains blood pH to 7.40, solidifies bones, and helps heal scars, and fight scurvy and germs. It is present in cartilage, fluids, and tissue. It is useful for Indigestion, headaches, muscle pains, arthritis, ileitis, colitis, asthma. Lack of calcium creates problems, symptoms, and disease in the areas mentioned above.

The one thing to remember is that calcium from food sources does not contribute to arteriosclerosis, calcium deposits, increase blood pressure, and other illnesses.

Calcium is one of the main minerals that promote healing in bones, tissue, organs, brain and in all parts of the body. It is carried to various parts of the body through the blood vessels. When you lack calcium, the infected or weaken areas do not get repaired properly and disease sets in. Without the necessary calcium your body needs, blood coagulation is affected and excess bleeding can occur.

Sun Glasses

Sunlight is a necessary energy that helps to ensure the absorptions of calcium. But, sunlight also plays another important role in regulating calcium throughout your body.

Sunlight or full-spectrum white light plays a major role in how the pituitary and pineal glands work. In the work place however, the lighting is artificial and this has a big impact on your long-term health.

The use of sunglasses is quite popular and because of the many different sunglass tints that exist, people wearing them filter out the sunlight frequencies associated with that tint. Full-spectrum light, like sun light, is necessary for proper function of the pituitary and pineal glands.

In the book, The Calcium Factor: The scientific Secret of Health and youth, 2000, Robert R. Barefoot & Carl J. Reich, M.D. say,

"When artificial full-spectrum lighting is used, human calcium absorption increases, plants flourish and cows produce 15% more milk...Tinted glasses can eliminate a large percentage of the sun's spectrum and therefore, affect you both physically and psychologically. Thus, full spectrum light plays a vital role in the maintenance of balanced hormonal system and is therefore indispensable in maintaining a balanced calcium serum."

Osteoporosis

Osteoporosis is the lack of calcium in the bone, and it is estimated that over 30% of the older population will develop this condition. This is not a condition that results from old age, but a condition that comes from having an acid body for a long time.

Since the endocrine glands exert a great amount of control over calcium, the endocrine glands are put out of balance by sugar. This causes an imbalance in calcium and then shows up as cavities in your teeth.

It is the imbalance of calcium in your body that is the start of the development of chronic illnesses.

Menstrual Flow

Menstrual blood contains up to 40 times more calcium than regular blood. If you have excessive flow, then you become depleted of calcium and iron. It is during this period that you should be eating kale, using liquid chlorophyll, and the many foods outlined in this e-book.

Without using a program that replaces your loss of calcium and iron during your periods, you open yourself to various diseases later. For a diet that contains plenty of iron you can check out my kindle e-book called, "Quick and Easy Diet Cures 4 Iron Deficiency Anemia."

Teeth health

Your teeth are made up of calcium phosphate. They

are kept healthy by your blood, and the nutrients that you supply them. The external part of your teeth is protected by enamel, which is an extremely strong material. But, acids that form in your mouth, when sugar is eaten, create an excess of bacteria that can penetrate that enamel.

Having dental cavities is a sign of lack of calcium. When your body needs calcium and you have not provided enough in your diet or your calcium body stores are depleted, calcium is pulled out of your teeth and bones to bring your body back into calcium balance. This weakens the teeth and bacteria can penetrate the enamel causing tooth decay.

Arteriosclerosis

Arteriosclerosis is not caused by an excess of calcium. It is caused by the lack of sodium and chlorine salts. Calcium needs these salts to be properly used and to stay in solution and not precipitate out onto artery walls. It is needed so that artery walls don't become inflamed by acid damage and consequently, need repair through plaque buildup.

Arteriosclerosis occurs when plaque builds up along the artery walls, which takes place over years. Eventually, this plaque will narrow the arteries and cause reduced blood flow or blood flow blockage. Reduced blood flow will result in many different illnesses because cells will not be getting the proper oxygen and nutrition. Blockage will result in heart attacks.

Plaque is made up of phospholipids, collagen, triglycerides, fibrin mucopolysaccharides, cholesterol, heavy metals, proteins, muscle tissue, and debris, which are all bonded by calcium.

Plaque only occurs in arteries that deliver blood from the heart to your body and not in the veins that return blood to the heart. Cholesterol is not the cause of plaque, but even if it was it can be controlled by diet and not drugs. Eighty percent of the cholesterol in your body is created in the body and 20% of it comes from your diet. Your body uses cholesterol in every cell, in hormones, in nerve impulses, in the brain, and in the creation of vitamin D on your skin.

It is the cellular breakdown along the artery walls caused by acidity surrounding the wall tissue or free radical damage that prompts repair of that area and that is when plaque starts to build up on the wall.

Heart Disease

Calcium is central to good heart function. Since calcium ions are linked to proper cell function, any deterioration you have in your cell do to the lack of calcium will affect the cell structure of heart cells and to the cells of the arteries. This deterioration will lead to heart diseases.

In addition the ability of the heart to contract and expand is due to the ionization of calcium, Ca++.

Effects Of Excess Calcium

When your body has an excess of calcium, you will see external and internal boney growths. These growths can occur in any part of your body such as joints, tissue, organs, or muscle. The growths may appear as kidney stones or other precipitates that occur on your heels, shoulder joints, knee joints, or toe bones.

When you have excess calcium, you need to eat more fruits and vegetables to get the natural absorbable vitamins and minerals, especially sodium. Sodium and calcium must always be in balance, lack of one or the other leads to a chemical imbalance, which results in various illnesses or diseases.

Illness or Conditions Due To Lack Of Calcium

Here some of the symptoms or conditions that occur when you lack calcium:

tumors
sores, abscesses, inflammations
discharges
deformed fingers, bones, hips cranial bones
tooth decay
undersized organs
blood deficiencies
back pain
vomiting
tuberculosis
excess bleeding
excess mucus discharge
poor scar healing

craving for salt
bone softening
swelling knuckles
bronchial congestion
wrinkled skin
cystic goiter
cyst formation
nervous problems

There are so many illnesses and poor body conditions that occur, when you lack calcium. You may have a few of these, but if they are consistent, and they remain with you for a while, consider increasing your calcium intake.

Nervous Problems

Anxiety is supposed to help you when you are involved in stressful or life-threatening situation. Under these conditions your metabolism increases, muscles tighten, and you get a shot of adrenaline. When anxiety happens, you use up many minerals, including calcium. Under stressful conditions that last more than a day, it is wise to take a calcium supplement.

Back pain

Back pain is one of those conditions that when it occurs, it can disable you and cause you to take a quick trip to emergency. When back pain is caused by strained muscles, stress, bad posture, in activity, or lack of exercise, one of the supplements recommend is calcium with magnesium. These minerals reduce muscle spasms, muscle tightness, and nerve irritation.

Taking a supplement that contains calcium, magnesium, and vitamin D daily, will help you to alleviate the long list of body conditions or illnesses. Just remember that calcium is a relaxer and nerve reliever.

Chapter 3: Eating The Best Calcium Foods

Even though you eat calcium foods, only around 25% of the calcium in this food will be absorbed by your body. But as a child or if you are pregnant, you may absorb up to 60%.

When cooking fruits or vegetables, you should use lower temperatures, when possible. When produce is heated to above 150 Fahrenheit, at least 33% of the available calcium is lost.

Calcium and Milk

All milk that is pasteurized at high temperatures is a low source of calcium. There is some milk that is pasteurized at 145 degrees Fahrenheit that are better sources of calcium. All milk that has been pasteurized or homogenized is acidic. The best milk source for calcium is raw goat milk and since it has not been heated it is alkaline in nature.

Despite the insistence from The Dairy Council that,

"Milk has been part of the diet for thousands of years. Despite the fact that milk is one of the most nutritionally complete foods available, there are many myths relating its consumption that blame milk and dairy foods for a variety of ailments. Many of these myths have been part of the folklore for centuries and are not founded on science."

There is a tremendous amount of scientific papers and finding that milk should not be included in your diet, because of the illnesses, it contributes too. But, there are studies that show there is a decrease in heart and cancer in people that drink milk.

An article, In 1992 The New England Journal of Medicine pointed out that, "Consumption of cow's milk has been associated with insulin-dependent diabetes..."

But, this is also evidence that some milk should be drunk and that there are other sources of dairy products that can provide plenty of calcium for your diet, such as yogurt or cottage cheese.

Because of the tremendous activity of calcium in the body in relation to cell nutrition and it alkalizing effect, it is best to eat plenty of those vegetables and fruits that are high in calcium.

In his book, **Prescription for Natural Cures**, 2004, by James F. Balch, M.D. he says,

"It may surprise you to learn that countries where people drink the most milk are also those with the highest rates of osteoporosis. This may be because lactose intolerance and casein allergy are very common and lead to mal-absorption. Also, calcium from cow's milk is not well absorbed, at a rate of 25 percent. Milk products lead to other health problems as well, so don't rely on them as source calcium. Unsweetened, cultured yogurt is an exception."

One way to eat your unsweetened yogurt is to add it to a blender and then add fruits like strawberries, pineapple, mango, bananas, and so on. To get additional sweetness, you can add some raw honey, since honey helps you to absorb calcium.

The British Medical Research Council made a 10-year study of 5000 men aged 45 to 59. In this study, they found, "only 1 percent of those who regularly drank more than one-half liter of milk a day suffered heart attacks ... against 10 per cent of those who drank no milk at all."
In this study, researchers also found there was no difference, whether they drank pure milk or skimmed, the benefits were still there.

There is still a lot of controversy about drinking milk for calcium. If you feel good drinking milk, then you should drink it. If you develop mucus or other symptoms, when you drink milk, then you should consider getting your calcium from other sources.

Where you can get calcium

One of the highest sources of calcium comes from **barley**, **green kale,** and **turnip greens**. You can get good calcium from cereals and grains.

Here is a list of foods highest in calcium:

Seaweed – dulse, kelp, Irish moss, wakame, nori, sombu, agar
Sardines with bones
Tempeh, tofu
Avocados, figs, prunes
All dark greens, collard greens, spinach, kale,
Unprocessed seeds and nuts – sesame seeds, grains, and nuts, almonds, walnuts
Bone broth
Cows, skimmed milk, cheese, cottage cheese, goat milk, yogurt
Rice milk-calcium enriched
Cabbage, cauliflower, celery, lemons, rhubarb
Egg yolk, gelatin foods
Fish, meat near the bone
Whole wheat bread
Beans, brown rice, lentils, millet, oats,
Broccoli, Brussels sprouts, cauliflower
Onions, parsnips, watercress
Raw butter, gelatin, blackstrap molasses
Coconut, raw cream, egg yolk
Fish, meat near the bone, bone broth
Natural cane sugar

The amount of calcium in certain foods

½ cup of wakame – sea vegetable gives 1700 mg
¼ cup of agar – sea vegetable gives 1000 mg
½ cup of nori – sea vegetable gives 600 mg
¼ cup of kombu – sea vegetable gives 500 mg
1 cup of tempeh gives 340 mg

8 oz. of calcium enriched rice milk give 300 mg
1 cup of almonds gives 300 mg
8 oz. of skim milk gives 302 mg
8 oz. of low fat yogurt gives 300 mg
1 oz. of Swiss cheese gives 272 mg
10 figs give 269 mg
½ cup of tofu gives 258 mg
½ cup of sesame seeds gives 250 mg
1 oz. of mozzarella cheese gives 183 mg
½ cup of boiled collards gives 179 mg
1 tablespoon of blackstrap molasses gives 172 mg
1 cup cottage cheese gives 126 mg
2 sardines in oil give 92 mg
¼ cup of walnuts gives 70 mg
1 cup of black beans or lentils gives 55 mg
½ cup of boiled mustard greens gives 52 mg
½ cup of boiled broccoli gives 36 mg

Dark Greens

The dark greens can be boiled instead of steamed, and their taste is improved. Boiling them also does not cause them to reduce their nutritional value, since they has such high nutrition to begin with.

Meat

Limit the amount of meat you eat. Meat has 30 times more phosphorous than calcium. And, in the digestive tract, this phosphorous will cause the calcium to precipitate to form apatite, which is a form of a phosphorous calcium mineral crystal. It is apatite that is the substance that forms your bones.

The result is that this calcium is not available to you and is excreted from your body.

Sugar

It has been found that there is 40% less calcium in white sugar as compared to raw sugar. Blackstrap molasses has 258 times more calcium as white sugar. Calcium and sugar attract each other. The more sugar you eat the more calcium is precipitated. The less body calcium you have the more tooth decay you will have.

Salt

Using excess salt in your food has been associated with bone loss. If you eat salt in your food, salt competes with calcium to get absorbed. The more salt is absorbed the less calcium is.

Try using culinary herbs and chili sauces to flavor your food. If you like salty food, you could use them as a snack and not with your regular meals.

Nightshades

Foods like tomatoes, potatoes, eggplant, peppers and tobacco, which are considered nightshade foods.

In her book, Food and Healing, 1986, Annemarie Colbin points out that,

"In my own experience and that of some of my

students, consuming nightshades on a dairy-free diet has resulted in a loss of calcium, evidenced by brittle nails, painful gums, and dental caries. Eliminating the nightshades, rather than increasing the dairy, solved the problem"

There are some foods that promote the excretion of calcium. We have indicated that eating excess meat can trap calcium and eliminate it from your body.

Foods high in oxalic acid also promote the removal of calcium from your body – spinach, cranberries, and rhubarb.

Wheat bran also limits the amount of calcium you absorb because to the phytic acid in its fiber. The phytic acid in wheat fiber has the ability to combine with calcium and limit its absorption in your body.

Other things that limit your calcium absorption are eating too many foods that contain phosphorus, drinking tea which contains tannins, lack of vitamin D, and having diarrhea.

Pumpkin Seeds

Shelled pumpkin seeds are a high source of zinc, magnesium, iron phosphorus, and calcium. You can eat a hand full every day.

Chapter 4: The Calcium Supplements You Should Take

Taking calcium supplements is a great idea, since you are probably not getting all the calcium you need in your diet.

However, since calcium tends to interfere with the absorption of other minerals, it is best to also take a multivitamin that provides those other minerals.

What type of calcium supplements should you take? A good supplement is one that contains:

Calcium 1000 – 1500 mg
Magnesium 400 – 600 mg
Vitamin D in Cholecalciferol form, called D3

So what are your daily requirements for calcium? Daily requirements for calcium are between 1000 to 1500mg. The type of supplement and the amount you take depends on your ability to absorb calcium. This is difficult to determine, so it is best to take the high end of calcium – 1500 mg.

Here are some minimum calcium supplementation requirements. Keep in mind that if you can get this amount in your food, then you don't need to take calcium supplements.

Infants 7-12 months   270 mg
Children 4-8 years   800mg
Males 31-50   1000mg
Females 31-50   1000mg
Pregnant and lactating 1000mg

One of the best calcium supplements to use is Brazil Live Coral.   It contains calcium, vitamin D, magnesium, and all the trace minerals.   It is in powder form so it is more absorbable. It contains the vitamin D you need to absorb the calcium.

But, you also need to spend at least 20 to 30 minutes in the sun to get the natural vitamin D. It does not have to be in the direct sunlight, but it is better, if you can do it. Look on the Internet for:

Brazil Live Coral

Also look for **Okinawa coral calcium** which is another good product.

Another excellent calcium supplement is called, **3-Way Calcium Complex™.** Look for this on the Internet. It uses three different forms of calcium and includes other nutrients that help you absorb more of this calcium.

Calcium absorption

For calcium to be absorbed in the body, it is crucial to have adequate vitamin D in your body. Without Vitamin D, calcium cannot be absorbed into your body. Vitamin D can be obtained from the sun and from supplements. Be aware that wearing sunglasses can affect your health by not keeping your pituitary gland healthy.

It's the pituitary gland that tells the parathyroid to release hormones that help to regulate and absorb calcium. In addition to eating calcium foods, take Brazil Live Coral Calcium and also add vitamin D as a supplement to your diet, especially if you don't go out into sun every day.

Vitamin C

It is believed that by taking vitamin C with Calcium, you increase the absorption of calcium. A form of calcium that is already combined with vitamin C is called Calcium Ascorbate. This type of calcium is easily transported across the intestinal walls.

Chelated calcium

It is best to use calcium supplements in chelated form. What this means is that calcium is tied to an amino acid and this makes it easier for calcium to pass through your intestinal walls. Chelated calcium is more easily absorbed than calcium that is not chelated. Here are some of the types of calcium amino acid chelates you should look for and buy.

Calcium Alpha Keto Glucarate
Calcium ascorbate – a form of calcium that is tied to vitamin C
Calcium Lactate
Calcium Arginate
Calcium hydroxyapatite – the type of calcium found in your bones
Calcium Glycinate
Calcium Amino Acid Chelate
Calcium Caprylate
Calcium Malate
Calcium Gluconate
Calcium L-Aspartate
Calcium Lactate Gluconate
Calcium Lysinate
Calcium Orotate
Calcium Succinate

Tri calcium phosphate – the type of calcium in your bones

All of these amino acids tied to calcium can also be attached to the other minerals like magnesium and potassium. So you can find magnesium arginate or magnesium alginate or magnesium aspartate.

Honey

It has been found by the United States Department of Agriculture nutritionist Richard J. Wood that the glucose in honey can increase your absorption of calcium by up to 25%. It can also increase the absorption of zinc and magnesium.

Types of Calcium to avoid

Calcium Dolomite

Avoid using dolomite as a source of calcium, since it may not be absorbed properly by your body. Dolomite is a form of calcium carbonate and magnesium.

Calcium carbonate

Calcium carbonate is hard to absorb when the pH in your stomach is not at the proper level. If you low levels of stomach acid you will not be able to absorb this type of calcium.

Magnesium

Magnesium is usually found in calcium supplements because it is required for proper calcium metabolism. Magnesium has a role in the formation of bones. It has been found that when there is a decrease in blood magnesium that there is also a drop in blood calcium. The lack of magnesium in your body can increase the risk of osteoporosis.

Magnesium's absorption is enhanced by vitamin D just like calcium is. Magnesium is active in making sure that cells function properly by moving sodium and potassium in and out of the cells. Magnesium, just like calcium, is important for nerve and heart function. Many of the foods that are high in calcium are also high in magnesium.

Chapter 5: How Calcium Makes You Alkaline

In this chapter, you will discover how you can make your body more alkaline. Calcium in addition to other minerals is one of the main minerals that can help you do this. Keeping your body alkaline is one of the best ways to keep your body calcium levels in balance.

Minerals

Moving your body more toward alkalinity is what will give you the best curative effects of fruits. An alkaline body prevents your body from becoming ill and forming deadly diseases, like all kinds of joint problems, organ degradation, body pain, or even cancer. If you are already sick, then all of the chemicals inside fruits will help to revive you to better health. This is provided that your tissue damage has not gone beyond repair.

The minerals most important in changing and maintaining your body in an alkaline condition are sodium, potassium, chloride, calcium, phosphorus, magnesium, and sulfur.

Now, how your body can become alkaline might become a little confusing at first because of the terms used, but let's break this down into small parts. This process has been discussed in previous chapters, but this explanation gives more details. First we are going to be defining some terms so we can then start talking the same language.

Acid Binding

There are certain minerals that are called acid binding. And these are minerals, as mentioned earlier, are the most important ones in fruits, Sodium, potassium, chloride, calcium, phosphorus, magnesium, because they are acid binding.

What acid binding means is when you eat fruits with these minerals, your cells, after metabolism, create an alkaline ash. This ash will seek out acids in your body and bind with them to neutralize them.

Alkaline Ash

Now, that this alkaline forming ash has tied up an acid it is carried to the kidney where it is expelled as urine.

Different reactions can occur when an acid binding mineral, like say sodium, encounters an acid. Of course, acids in the body are toxic, so the body has the priority of getting rid of them fast, since they can damage tissue and cause pain and disease.

Here is another path way of the acid binding mineral process when it combines with an acid.

The Acid Binding Mineral Process

When you eat acid binding food, the blood carries it to the cells where it is oxidized, digested, or metabolized. The result of this digestion is a carbonic acid salt of alkaline minerals, which reacts with body acids and binds with them. In this process, a weak carbonic acid is created. Now, this weak carbonic acid is taken by the blood into the lungs where it is released as carbon dioxide and water.

If not all the acid toxins are captured by acid binding matter, the remaining acids can be neutralized by body stores of alkaline minerals. If you don't have a good store of alkaline minerals, then these acids will remain in your body creating pain and disease.
But if you do have a good store of alkaline minerals, then these minerals will find these acids, capture them and bind with them. Then these acids are routed out through your urine or colon and out of your body.

So you can see the importance of getting a lot of alkaline minerals into your body. Without them, acids which do not get bonded to alkaline minerals would move back into body tissue and continue their body damage.

Alkaline Binding

Now, there are also minerals that become alkaline binding and these minerals are sulphur, chlorine, iodine, phosphorous, bromine, fluorine, copper, and silicon.

It is these minerals that when digested by a cell will produce an acid salt that will bind with alkaline minerals. These minerals will be excreted through your urine. When alkaline minerals are bonded to an acid salt, the alkaline mineral is removed from your body, and your body becomes more acidic, the condition you are trying to avoid. Although you need to eat both foods that are acid binding and alkaline binding, you want to eat more of the acid binding food.

Keeping Healthy

One of the most important parts of health is keeping the lymph liquid around your cells clean and free of toxins. To do this you need provide alkaline minerals to occupy the lymph liquid and you need to remove the acids that accumulate in that liquid and in all parts of your body tissue. You can do this by detoxifying your body and providing alkaline minerals for your lymph liquid.

Body Detoxification

The highest priority of the body is to detoxify itself. One of the
best way to help your body detoxify is to provide minerals that bind with acids that are in the cells, tissues, organs, and muscles. What these alkaline acid binding minerals do is to pull out the toxins that are dispersed throughout your body.

With the help of the liver which detoxifies the blood, the kidney that removes impurities from the blood and the lungs which removes the CO_2 which results from alkaline acid binding, your body is constantly detoxifying itself. But when it is over loaded with acid toxins from your lifestyle, a complete detox of your body becomes impossible.

Where do Acid Toxins Come From

So why is the body overloaded with toxins? Why can't the liver take care of these toxins? The liver has the function to remove acid wastes from natural food that is created by food digestion and cell metabolism. When it encounters acid wastes such as food enhancers, dyes, preservatives, pesticides, and the variety of additives, the liver does not always know how to break them down to make them harmless.

But your body does not give up so easily when it knows that the liver was not able to disintegrate food additives. What it does is it instructs calcium to bind with these toxic acids and to take them far away from the blood stream.

The result is that calcium binding with acid forms a deposit and this deposit can be placed in your teeth, your joints, and as bone spurs, which grow in your feet or shoulders, vertebra, or muscle tissue. These calcium deposits are very painful, and if you have ever experience them, you know how much.

Now, we have talked about acid toxins in the body

that are brought in through food and the environment. But, there are another factors that creates acid in the body and those are emotions that are occur through life stresses, like work pressures, divorce, friendship problems, martial issues, and other similar problems. These emotional problems create acidic molecules that embed themselves into your tissues just like food acids.

Body Organs

All body organs function to rid the body of acid waste or toxins. Lack of alkaline binding food causes deterioration of the function of these organs. Each organ has a specific function in the elimination and neutralization of acid wastes and it does this in conjunction with alkaline acid binding minerals.

Here is the list of the fruits that have the highest alkaline minerals and the ones that you should be eating. The percentage number next to them indicates the strength of the alkaline mineral and the closer to 100% the more effective it is as an acid binding fruit. However, you should be eating all of these fruit not just the ones at the top of the list.

The percentage assigned to these fruits is based on fresh fruits that are organic and that they are not cooked, canned or mixed with sugar. If they are cook or otherwise processed in some fashion, this will reduce their effectiveness as an acid binding. However, they will still be effective in acid binding.

Acid Binding Fruits With Alkaline Minerals

In the list below are fruits with alkaline minerals that create an acid binding salt your body uses to neutralize acid wastes.

Fruits above 50% in value are more acid binding, which means they will more trap acid wastes.

Here is the list of fruits to eat in the order of priority.

Fruits at 100% Acid Binding – Best fruits To Eat Lemons, melons – any type, watermelon
Fruits at 93% Acid Binding – Great fruits To Eat Cantaloupes, dried dates, dried figs, limes, mango,
papaya

Fruits at 87% Acid Binding – Still Great Fruits To Eat Kiwis, passion fruit, pineapples, raisins, umeboshi plums

Fruits at 80% Acid Binding – Eat These Fruits Apricots, avocados, bananas, fresh dates, fresh figs, currants, gooseberries grapes, grapefruits guavas, kumquats, nectarines, pears, persimmons, quince

Fruits at 73% Acid Binding – Still Fruits To Eat Apples, organs, peaches, pomegranate, raspberries, sour grapes, strawberries

Fruits at 67 Acid Binding – Still Neutralizes Acids
        Cherries

Fruits To Concentrate On

These are the fruits you should concentrate on eating. Also eat them every day, if possible, fresh lemon juice in the morning, watermelon during the day.

You can see which fruits give you the best acid binding effects and eating them 80% of your overall food intake will convert your body over to an Alkaline body.

NOW LET'S GO TO THE NEXT SECTION ON MAGNESIUM MAGIC

Section 2: Magnesium Magic

Chapter 6: Why You Need Magnesium

Half of the magnesium you have in your body is found in your bones and the other half is in your soft tissue. It is found in your skeletal muscles, liver, heart and pancreas.

Magnesium is considered a "forgotten mineral." Most people don't think about magnesium like they do calcium, potassium or iron. Almost 90% of the population may be short on magnesium, since it has been found that they only consume about 40% of the daily recommended requirement.

If you are short in magnesium, you may not show any symptoms, you may just ignore them, or you may attribute them to some other nutrient deficiency. However, moderate or severe magnesium deficiency results in malnutrition, loss of appetite, nausea, weakness, personality changes and arrhythmias.

Magnesium in Chlorophyll

Magnesium is a major mineral like sodium, calcium, and potassium. It is central to the food chain in that it holds a position in chlorophyll, the blood of plants. It appears in the center of the chlorophyll molecule. Chlorophyll is similar to the hemoglobin molecule except that at the center of the hemoglobin molecule is the mineral iron.

So, if you want to build your blood, drinking chlorophyll is one ways to do. It's the magnesium in the chlorophyll that also
helps make white blood cells that fight infection and which combines with red blood cells.

When your body is low in hemoglobin, drinking chlorophyll will help increase the hemoglobin in your blood. Your body has the power to transmute or to transform magnesium into iron, which helps to make more hemoglobin. It does this through multiple chemical changes that start with oxygen.

Magnesium Requirements

The overall balance of minerals in your body's lymph liquids, outside your cells and inside your cells, determines your health. When your minerals are balanced similar to sea water, you will have better health.

The sea has a high level of magnesium, so that water inside your cells should also be high in magnesium, since magnesium is used to transport nutrients in and out of your cells. Magnesium is a major mineral that is needed in the right quantities, so that you can achieve maximum health.

Most people ignore the importance of magnesium. It is important to know what magnesium does in your body. You need to know what foods to eat to get the maximum magnesium in your body. You should know what symptoms you will have, when you don't get the proper amount of magnesium.

If you know how magnesium is regulated in your body, then you can help your body maintain and keep the amount that your body needs. Also, if you know what illnesses need more magnesium, you can help yourself get well.

Magnesium and Enzymes

Magnesium is involved in activating over 300 different enzymes and body chemicals. It helps to active the B vitamins.

It works in protein synthesis, muscle excitability and helps to release energy. In your cells, it converts fat, carbohydrates, and protein into the energy your body needs. It helps to regulate blood sugar, nerve impulses, and electrical potential across cell walls. And, it tones brain blood vessels and keeps them relaxed and open, so that nutrients can get into your brain cells.

Magnesium and Bones

You will find magnesium mostly in your cells, in the mitochondria, which is the energy center of your cells. Magnesium regulated the absorption of calcium and maintains the construction of bones and teeth. Lack of magnesium can lead to brittle bones and osteoporosis. Your parathyroid gland also needs magnesium to regulate your blood calcium levels.

Magnesium is the third most important nutrient in building bones, after calcium and vitamin D. Half of all the magnesium in your body is found in your bones. When you lack magnesium, you are susceptible to forming calcium crystals in your bones and in other body locations.

Stress

If you are constantly under stress because of your job, you home life, or your regular life, then most likely, you will be low on magnesium. The same holds true if you stress your body physically by doing exercise and playing sports.

Chapter 7: The Magic of the Mineral Magnesium

"A mineral that relaxes the body – magnesium"

Like sodium, calcium, and potassium, magnesium also has a positive charge and is represented by the symbol, Mn+. Because of this, magnesium helps to make your body more alkaline. Your bones hold up to 60% of the body's magnesium, and the extracellular liquid contains around 1%.

Your body holds up to 3 oz. of magnesium. It is alkaline in nature and it is known as the "Relaxer", since helps to calm the nerves and muscle tissue. But, calming the nerve is also a matter of mind control and attitude. You can increase your life span, when you are calmer and have the proper amount of magnesium in your body.

In your body, magnesium takes the form of:

Magnesium carbonate
Magnesium silicate
Magnesium chloride
Magnesium sulphate (Epsom salt)
Magnesium phosphate.

When you have plenty of magnesium in your body,

you have good motion and can do many physical activities. Here is a list of what magnesium does in your body.

Alkalinizes the body
Produces laxative action
Calms the nerves
Keeps the body flexibly
Influences glands
Combats acids and toxins
Eliminates poisons
Prevents deposition of phosphates in joints
Neutralizes phosphoric acid
Promotes carbohydrate metabolism in the cells
Helps produce and use body energy
Helps in DNA and protein creation
Assists Potassium and sodium cross cell membrane during Potassium – Sodium Pump action
Regulates muscle movements
Helps maintain calcium levels in the extracellular fluid

Magnesium does its work by reducing tension, relaxing your body, and improving bowel movements. It reduces nerve irritation by neutralizing the chemicals or by-products that are created when your body is going through tense and irritable conditions.

Your body regulates the amount of magnesium it retains and stores by using the gastrointestinal tract, GI tract, and urinary system. If you need more magnesium in your body, the GI tract will absorb more in the small intestine. If your body has too much magnesium, the GI tract will excrete some of it and eliminate it through your stools.

Your kidneys are also involved in controlling the amount of magnesium your body retains. If magnesium levels fall, the kidneys closely control how much magnesium goes into your urine. Similarly, if the magnesium levels are too high, the kidneys will excrete more through your urine.

Regulation of Magnesium

Many things control how much magnesium and calcium you absorb. If magnesium in your body goes up, calcium stores will go down and if magnesium stores fall, then calcium body stores go up. Your stomach absorbs a lot of magnesium for hydrochloric acid production, HCl. When you take in food or calcium supplements, protein, vitamin D, or alcohol, your body needs more magnesium. And, caffeine, sugar, phosphorus, excess sodium, diuretics, and alcohol increase the loss of magnesium through urine.

You will increase the amount of magnesium you absorb, when you drink milk, because of the presence of lactose.

Magnesium as a laxative

Magnesium has natural laxative powers. When you eat foods that have magnesium your regularity improves. When magnesium is consumed and reaches your blood, some of it is transported into your colon walls. Where it softens your stools and helps to produce peristaltic action. For this reason fruits and vegetables that contain some or are high in magnesium promote regularity – yellow and winter squashes, grapefruits, apricots, oranges, peaches, and corn.

Chapter 8: The Best Magnesium Foods

Here is a list of the foods that you should eat to get plenty of magnesium:

Best foods with magnesium:

Rice bran, pumpkin seeds, wheat germ, sunflower seeds, sesame seeds, seaweed agar, cashews, hazelnuts, fermented soy products

Other great foods for magnesium:

Peanuts	leafy greens	seeds
Buckwheat	bananas	beet greens
Oats	avocados	black-eyed peas
Baked potato	with skins	blackstrap
molasses		
Cabbage,	dandelion	brown rice
Rice bran,	pomegranates	barley
Whole wheat	walnuts	mustard greens
Almonds	nuts	rye
Nettles	chestnuts	berries
Seafood	green leafy	vegetables
Dry beans and peas		meat

Chocolate

Many people crave chocolate. This may be because they are deficient in magnesium. Chocolate, especially cocoa, has a high concentration of magnesium. In one cup of unsweetened cocoa, you have 400 mg of magnesium and 2159 mg of potassium. It also has many other minerals, but in smaller quantity. Cocoa is also known for is high level of antioxidants.

To get the best benefits of cocoa, you need to eat chocolate that has at least 85% cocoa.

However when you eat chocolate candy, which has bittersweet chocolate, or semisweet baking chocolate, it has up to 65% sugar and a fat level of 20 – 35%. Cocoa has 2% sugar and has a fat level of up to 15%. Using unsweetened or bittersweet chocolate in cooking is ok, since its sugar level is 2 – 45%.

What is not good about chocolate is it is also high in caffeine and theobromine, which stimulate the adrenals that can lead to adrenal fatigue.

Yellow Cornmeal

Yellow cornmeal, high in magnesium, has excellent laxative powers. Use it 3 or 4 times a week and improve your regularity. Cornmeal, cooked slowly under low heat, can easily be use with children or adults that are constipated. Or, you can prepare raw corn soup by:

1 ½ cups raw corn off the cob
Vegetable broth to taste

2 bay leaves
1 ½ cup of raw milk, cream, or milk
Put all this into a blender and warm slightly

Calms the Nerves

Magnesium is a relaxer of nerves. When you are tense, nervous, get irritated, or turn hot tempered, you develop ulcers, colitis, constipation, and colon spastic conditions. Magnesium will help to reduce or minimize these conditions. It enters the nerve fibers, with the help of albumin and water.

When you first take magnesium for nerves or for any other condition, you will have to use it for a month or more to see results. It takes that long and even longer for magnesium to fill your body reserves, so that it is available to constantly serve your body's needs.

If you have lower-back problems, you need to have plenty of magnesium. When you are tense, any adjustments a chiropractor gives will go out of adjustment, when your body is low in magnesium. The adjustment will be made and your tense ligaments or muscles will pull back the adjustment to its previous position.

Magnesium is found in tendons, ligaments, tissue, joints, and nerves and helps them to relax and to maintain bones in position.

Cramps in your calves, at night, call for magnesium and calcium, which prevents the stiffening of tissue and muscle due to excess acids.

Alkalizes the body

Magnesium combines with acids, gases, waste, impurities, and toxins to clean your body and make your body more alkaline. Magnesium sulphate pulls toxic buildup and waste from your intestinal walls and eliminates them through your stools.

A good supply of magnesium is necessary to make your body alkaline and to combine with poisons and heavy metals. Magnesium has the ability to combine with poisons that create diseases. It combines with excess albumin, lead, phosphorus, chloride, antimony, ferrous sulphate, barium, muriatic acid, uric acid, urate acid, and ptomaine.

In the brain, magnesium combines with phosphoric by products that occur when you do excessive mental work.

Chapter 9: Deficiency And Excesses Of Magnesium

Deficiencies of Magnesium

When you become dehydrated, you lose magnesium. When you take calcium you will deplete your stores of magnesium. Drinking too much milk also will deplete your body's magnesium.

Young athletes who drink too much milk need to be careful, since they tend to lose magnesium. Retired and geriatric people should always take a magnesium supplement.

If you are taking diuretics of any kind, natural remedies or drugs, you will slowly lose your magnesium. The more diuretics you use the more magnesium you lose.

When you are deficient in magnesium, you are over sensitive about everything in your life. You are hyperactive, anxious, fidgety, energetic, mentally active, and industrious. There are so many symptoms when you are deficient in magnesium that it is hard to tell when you are deficient.

The more serious symptoms are muscle spasms and seizures. There is now some evidence that magnesium deficiency has an important role in many heart ailments. Dr. Alexander Heggtveit, at the University of Ottawa in Canada, found fatal attack victims with less magnesium than those that died of other causes.

You can have a magnesium deficiency after prolonged diarrhea and vomiting or with long term laxative and diuretic use. If you frequently drink too much alcohol then, you will be deficient in magnesium.

Elderly people are at high risk for magnesium deficiency, since they absorb it poorly. If they supplement with too much calcium or use too many drugs, this can deplete their magnesium body stores.

When you have a low level of magnesium, you will have an increase in calcium blood levels, which contribute to the formation of kidney stones. If the low levels continue, magnesium will be pulled out of the heart muscles, causing a disruption in its function.

When your blood levels of magnesium are low, your body takes magnesium that is stored in your tissues, which leads to muscle weakness, fatigue, irritability and nervousness.

Here is a list of symptoms you can have when you have a low level of magnesium.

Head tremors
Voice breaks or stammers
Unclear conversations
Feeling of doom
Smelly feet
Muscles are weak
Constipation
Poor kidney function
Poor sleep
Back pain
Heart palpitations
Eyelids twitch
Osteoporosis
High blood pressure
Migraine headaches
Appetite for acid food and drink
Nausea
Heavy head in morning
Shoulder and neck muscles tense at night

Hypomagnesemia

A deficiency in magnesium is called Hypomagnesemia. This deficiency is when the amount of your body's magnesium falls below 1.8mEq/L. The unit mEq/L is a measure given to the amount of substance in a body per liter. This deficiency can occur when you:

don't eat enough magnesium foods
have poor absorption of magnesium in GI tract
have excess magnesium loss in GI tract
have excess magnesium loss in urinary tract – kidney

use excess coffee, alcohol, sugar, and tobacco

Negative emotions also deplete magnesium that is in reserves and in intracellular liquid. If you constantly live these emotions below, then you will be short of magnesium:

Hatred, resentment, jealousy, quarrels, bitterness, temper outbursts, selfishness, greed fear, panic, worry, paranoia, overwork, over study, loss of love one.

Other symptoms you can have with low magnesium are:

Cardiac arrhythmias
Digoxin toxicity
Laryngeal strid or Respiratory muscle weakness
Seizures
Arthritis deformans
Poor elimination
Over excitement
Nervous headaches
Ulcers
Acute diarrhea
Eyes tearing excessively or excess catarrh of eye lens
Nosebleeds
Sex brain nerve ends and nerve fiber irritation
Decrease in electrical nerve impulses
Extreme colitis
Urine retention
Sleeplessness, fainting
Hot temper, forgetfulness

Drastic mood changes
Increase in asthmatic attacks
Free Radical Damage

When you are magnesium deficient, the body starts taking magnesium out of your cells. As you reduce cell magnesium, your muscles grow weak and nerves and muscles become highly irritable.

Free Radical Damage

Low levels of magnesium can magnify the damage caused by free radicals. It has also been seen that it can start the production of free radicals.

Excess of Magnesium

You can have excess magnesium in your body, when you eat an excess of magnesium foods, supplements, tonics or drugs. When you have an excess of magnesium in your body, the sedative effects of magnesium are intensified. Your memory decreases, you become less active, and do not have good reasoning skills. Your nerve endings become less sensitive and depressed and your perception and intelligence is decreased. You become less interested in life and you sleep more.

Hypermagnesemia

Excessive magnesium in your body is called Hypermagnesemia. This condition occurs when you have a magnesium level above 2.5 mEq/L. This condition is rare, since kidneys can quickly remove excess magnesium. But when it does occur, and the cause could be:

Kidney dysfunction
Addison's disease
Adrenocortical insufficiency
Excess use of antacids or laxatives
Excess use of magnesium rich dialysate
Excess use of TPN solutions
Excess use of magnesium sulfate in treating seizures, or hypertension

Patellar Reflex

If your patellar reflex, the tapping just below the knee to see if the leg extension occurs, is absent, it's an indication that your magnesium level is 7 mEq/L or higher. This high level makes your nerves relax creating an absence of leg reflex in the patellar test.

Magnesium Laxative

Excess magnesium is quickly removed, from your body by the onset of diarrhea. But, one of the issues is that you can develop an excess of magnesium when you use a large amount over-the-counter, drugstore products, for acid reflux or constipation. Overdose on magnesium is a rare occurrence.

Large amounts of magnesium can be toxic. You can end up with excess magnesium, if you have kidney disease or if your calcium body levels are low and your phosphorus intake is high.

Chapter 10: The Best Magnesium Supplements

Taking Magnesium Supplements

Do not take magnesium supplements if you have kidney weakness or disease. Also if you have heart problems, do not take more than 350 mg of magnesium. It is always safe to see your doctor about what dose you should take.

Fast Magnesium

If you have gut spasms or other body conditions where you need to receive magnesium fast, you can do it as follows:

Buy a Magnesium Chloride Solution 18%, Ecologic Formulas Brand, on the Internet or at a health food store. Add 1-2 teaspoons to a glass of water and drink twice a day. The taste is not too good, but you will get magnesium into your body quickly.

It is estimated that a typical American diet provides only around 30% to 50% of the 500 mg of the daily requirements for magnesium. In addition, around 80% of the diets eaten in American are magnesium deficient.

Magnesium is easier to lose than other minerals and especially when you eat or take an increase in calcium. When you supplement with magnesium you should check that the supplement has equal amounts of magnesium and calcium. If it has more calcium, you will lose some magnesium. Or, it would be better to take magnesium as a separate supplement and taken when you don't take calcium.

Magnesium Citrate

Use a magnesium citrate supplement. Take this supplement after 8pm with vitamin C and pantothenic acid, since these three nutrients work together. Always take magnesium and all other minerals and trace minerals with tomato juice or apple juice or at meals with whole grapes, meat or digestive enzymes.

This provides acid to dissolve and absorb the magnesium quicker. You can also take it after 8pm or just before bedtime without any food.
.

There are other forms of magnesium that are also good, since they are tied to an amino acid or are so called "chelated." and these are,

Magnesium citrate
Magnesium gluconate,
Magnesium Aspartate
Magnesium taurate

Magnesium oxide – avoid using this type, because it is not as absorbable as the other types.

Magnesium and Calcium Supplements

Look for a combination supplement of calcium, magnesium, vitamin D and with a 1:1 ratio of calcium to magnesium. This type of ratio is hard to find, but you should be able to find it on the Internet. Most ratios your will find are 2:1 with calcium being twice as much as magnesium.

Here is other some other magnesium combinations that you should consider, if you can't fine the supplements above:

Potassium- magnesium citrate
Magnesium citrate – potassium- taurine

Taking too much magnesium can cause diarrhea, lethargy or weakness. This mineral can also interfere with any antibiotic you might be taking, so it best not to supplement with it when taking antibiotics or even other drugs.

How Much Magnesium?

Some doctors and nutritionists say that, you should have twice as much magnesium as calcium in your supplement. This will insure that you will have strong bones. Most supplements that contain these minerals are of the opposite ratio; they have twice as much calcium as magnesium. But, taking a supplement with a 1:1 ratio should be where you can start.

Daily magnesium supplementation is:

Children to 14 years, 270 mg
Males 15 and older, 500 mg
Males 51 years and older 600 mg
Females 15 and older, 300 mg
Females 51 years and older 550 mg

In some cases, for adults, up to 1200 mg is recommended. Over dosing is very hard with magnesium, since the kidney and the colon will excrete the excess. If you start to exhibit signs of diarrhea or body weakness, back off on the amount, you are taking.

Vitamin D

You need the proper levels of magnesium to activate the vitamin D your body needs. If you have a magnesium deficiency, then you will have lower levels of vitamin D. Make sure you have the Vitamin D3 type of supplement.

B vitamins

When you take Vitamin B6, you improve the intake of magnesium into your cells. You can supplement with a vitamin B 50 or B100 to get the needed B vitamins.

Copper

Because magnesium is easily lost in the urine, when you are dehydrated, you can take three mg of copper, and this will stop the loss of magnesium in your urine.

Over The Counter Magnesium Products

Magnesium toxicity can occur with individuals with kidney failure. Toxicity effects have been found in some individuals that use laxative such as Epsom salts, magnesium sulfate and milk of magnesia, or magnesium hydroxide. These laxatives are typically used at 3,000 to 5,000 mg per day. Toxic effects have been found when these laxatives are used at 9,000 mg per day.

If you have a deficiency of magnesium, it will take around 6 months of magnesium supplementation to get your body back to normal levels of magnesium. Your body uses magnesium every day, so you need to supply it with this amount every day. Any excess can go to neutralize acids. Then if still have some left over, this will go to various body areas to be store.

Chapter 11: Illnesses Eliminated With Magnesium

There are certain illnesses that you can reduce, eliminate and even cure, if you increase your intake of magnesium. Some of these illnesses are caused by the lack of magnesium.

These illnesses are:

Cardiovascular
Chronic fatigue syndrome
Kidney stones
Muscle cramps
Preeclampsia – during pregnancy
Osteoporosis
PMS symptoms
Migraines
Respiratory disease
Alzheimer's disease
Back problems
Free Radicals
Migraines
Digestive Problems
Eye problems
Constipation

Cardiovascular

Having a low level of magnesium can result in more blood clots. It has been found that women that use oral contraceptives have lower levels of magnesium. This is the reason why there is a higher occurrence of thrombosis in women who use these contraceptives.

A deficiency of magnesium can damage the arteries in the heart, which results in plaque buildup. High blood pressure is also associated with a magnesium deficiency. There is a tendency for those with diabetes and low magnesium to have more cardiovascular issues.

So keep your levels of magnesium high by eating and supplementing with the suggestions given here. Magnesium helps to reduce the possibility of you having a heart attack, stroke, angina, or heart surgery. Eating nuts of various kinds every work day will help you stop heart attacks.

Kidney Stones

If you have kidney stones, you can get rid of them by using 1000 mg of magnesium citrate and 100 mg of B6. If you just want to make sure you don't accumulate stones, you can use this supplement combination on occasion for a week. Kidney stones are a combination of calcium and oxalic acid. When these two combine in the kidney, they form calcium oxalate crystals.

To minimize the amount of oxalic acid you have in your body, avoid eating cooked spinach or other green tops. Eat them raw when possible.

Muscle Cramps

Magnesium helps to relax muscle and without it you are prone to muscle cramps. When calcium moves into muscle tissue, your muscles will contract. When calcium leaves the muscles, and magnesium moves into your muscles, your muscles will relax. Excess deficiency of magnesium leads to muscle spasms, tremors, and convulsions. If you have leg cramps at night, take a combination of calcium, magnesium, and vitamin D. This will put an end to these cramps. Take this supplement just before bedtime.

Osteoporosis

To have strong bones and teeth you need minerals. It's calcium that makes bones strong in conjunction with other minerals such as phosphorous, magnesium, strontium, silica, zinc, copper, and boron. Magnesium is definitely needed to prevent osteoporosis.

PMS symptoms

There are some women that crave chocolate before their period or who have PMS. It is known that magnesium helps resolve the symptoms of PMS, since it is involved in the production of progesterone. A lack of magnesium can produce decreased progesterone levels resulting in PMS symptoms.

It's better to avoid chocolate, since it creates adrenal fatigue. It is better to eat those foods that are high in magnesium or to take 400 mg of magnesium citrate. Take this magnesium with some vitamin C and B6 just before bedtime. Magnesium is absorbed better after 8pm. This combination of nutrients will help to reduce the intensity and duration of PMS.

Pregnancy

Magnesium has a powerful influence in the prevention of pregnancy complication, such as prematurity and intrauterine growth retardation.

Migraines

There are studies that show magnesium can prevent or relieve migraines. By using high doses of 1000 mg or more, magnesium was shown to be just as effective as established drugs, such as flunarizine and amitriptyline.

Respiratory Disease

Magnesium has been found to be helpful in respiratory disease such as bronchitis and asthma. Eat those foods that are high in magnesium, but you need to be aware of those foods that you might be allergic to, which aggravate your respiratory condition.

Alzheimer's Disease

Having a low level of magnesium and calcium in your body opens you up to toxic aluminum deposit in your brain nerve cells. When you have these low levels of these minerals, your body will accept the use of other minerals in their place. So if you also have an excess of aluminum, your body will use it in place of magnesium or calcium and when these minerals reach your brain they deposit in your brain cells.

The result is that you have the onset of senility, or you develop Alzheimer's. Under these conditions, zinc is the recommend mineral to prevent senile changes in your brain.

Magnesium is involved in keeping your brain cells alive. It does this by reducing the negative effects of less blood flow to the brain and by insuring that nutrients reach your brain cells. It also prevents the buildup of calcium in your brain cells, which is associated with Alzheimer's.

Back Problems

Magnesium will help you build a strong straight back. It aids in the inter-vertebral structure. It is in this structure where magnesium is stored. It is also stored in the colon. If the vertebral structure and colon don't get enough magnesium, they will not function properly.

Free Radicals

It has been seen by researchers that low levels of magnesium give way to free radical formation thus exposing cells to more radical attack.

Migraines

It has been found that 50% of people with migraines have magnesium deficiency. You can get some relief by taking 400+ mg of magnesium daily with meals.

Digestive Problems

If you have stomach problems such as vomiting, cramps, indigestion, flatulence, stomach pain, or constipation, all this could be related to low levels of magnesium.

Eye problems

If you are diabetic, you will want to keep high levels of blood magnesium. If you do, you are less likely to develop diabetic retinopathy. In addition, if you have glaucoma, it will lessen the effects of this condition.

Constipation

Magnesium is hydrophilic and likes water. In your colon it will draw water and make your stools soft. Magnesium is used in many over-the-counter laxatives. Using these laxative, gives you high levels of magnesium salts. If you are deficient in magnesium, you will have constipation.

Sweaty Hands

Have you ever shaked hands with someone who has sweaty hands or that has excess body order? Aside from not showering frequently, this person may be deficient in magnesium. The use of liquid chlorophyll will help reduce the body order.

Chapter 12: Final Magnesium Comments

In your cells, tissues, muscles, and nerves, magnesium neutralizes acids, toxic matter, and wastes that are created when you become anxious, nervous, hot tempered, over excited, or overworked. It helps to neutralize those acids that come from eating too much acid food. Use magnesium foods and supplements to help get your body alkaline.

When you eat a lot of meat and other acid foods with little vegetables, you will deplete your stores of magnesium and you will need to use all the information listed in this book to restore your magnesium body levels. Magnesium is known as the "Relaxer" since it calms your nervous and muscular system.

You can have an under or over supply of magnesium in your body. Your kidney and colon are responsible for maintaining the proper magnesium balance in your body. It will excrete excessive magnesium into your urine or it will stop excreting it when your body supplies are low. And, with under supplies, magnesium will be pulled out of your cells to satisfy your body's needs. When it does this your body will be acidic and prone to disease.

Eat Magnesium Foods

Eat magnesium foods daily. Use seeds in your smoothies and nuts as midday snacks. Eat a variety of vegetables. Choosing 4 or 5 vegetable properly can give you plenty of all the minerals you need. However, by choosing a variety of fruits and vegetables, you get certain nutrients and antioxidants that are only available in each fruit or vegetable.

Magnesium Supplements

When you buy a magnesium supplement it is best to buy it with calcium and vitamin D. Calcium needs magnesium and vitamin D to complete its digestion and absorption into your body. Choose those supplements that are tied to an amino acid, like Magnesium Citrate. This allows this mineral to be pulled through your intestinal wall easier and faster. Look for a magnesium supplement that has just as much magnesium as calcium, 1:1.

If you have a lot of anxiety and stress in your life you will need to take up to 1000 mg of magnesium. Stress uses up a lot of magnesium.

Look at the list of illnesses and body conditions listed in the previous chapters and see if you have some of these symptoms or diseases. If so, then you too should be taking up to 1000 mg of magnesium. If you have issues with your kidney or heart, then talk to your doctor about how much magnesium you should take.

Excess Magnesium

If you take too much magnesium, you will get diarrhea. Just back off on the amount you are taking, until your diarrhea goes away.

Chapter 13: About The Author And Other Resources

Get one of my best kindle books *free* below:

http://www.natural-remedies-thatwork.com

Rudy Silva is a natural nutritional consultant educated in the United States in Nutrition and Physics. He is a graduate from San Jose State University in California. He is author of 45 other books on natural remedies. He has authored a newsletter in natural remedies for over 10 years.

Resource page

Here are some of the other kindle e-books about natural remedies that have been written by this author. You can see the entire list at:

http://tinyurl.com/b2f7wd3

Acne Remedies
- Best natural acne treatments: Acne facial
- Effective Acne Treatments That Work

Constipation Remedies
- The Best Constipation Remedies
- Best Constipated Women Natural Cures
- How To Relieve Constipation With Fruits

Essential Fatty Acids
- Taking The Mystery Out Of Essential Fatty acids
- Amazing Fish Oil Benefits Revealed
- Omega 3 and 6 Mystery Exposed

Nutrition Remedies
- Updated Version - Secret Diet And Nutrition
- Secret Healthy Fruit Practices Revealed
- Fast Healing Juice Nutrition Therapy: Nutrition Tips 3
- Fantastic Alkaline Fruit Benefits Revealed
- Calcium (Discover How To Use Calcium To Avoid Devastating Diseases)
- Magnesium Nutrition Revealed
- Best Nutrition Health Practices
- Potassium Health Secrets Revealed
- Phosphorus, The Best Brain Food
- A Sodium Diet (What You Must Know About Sodium)
- Vegetables and Vegetable Juice Cures
- Alkaline Body: How to Change an Acid Body into an Alkaline body

Stomach Remedies
- Acid Reflux: Fast and Easy Cures For Acid Reflux
- Asthma Treatment Cures With Remedies
- How To Do Natural Colon Cleansing
- Gastrointestinal Digestion Secrets Revealed

Misc Remedies
- Natural Hair Loss Treatment: Women And Men
- Effective Natural Hemorrhoids Treatment
- Iron Deficiency Anemia
- Secrets To Understanding Behavior
- Fast Acting Ear Infection Remedies
- Best Behavior Secrets Revealed That Can Change Your Personality
- What Is A Hiatus Hernia
- Best Varicose Vein Treatments?
- Make Shampoos At Home Using Natural Ingredients:Discover recipes for quality natural hair shampoos
- How To Fix Your Thyroid Problems: Discover Hidden Ideas That Fix Your Thyroid

Minerals
- Calcium and Magnesium Magic Body Benefits Revealed
- The Magic of Sodium, Calcium and Magnesium
- Create an Alkaline Body with Potassium and Sodium: Eliminate a Potassium Deficiency

- Calcium and Phosphorus Foods: Deficiency or Excesses in These Minerals Cause Bone and Brain Power Loss
- Chlorine The Body Detoxifier (With water, chlorine will clean your body of toxins and pathogens)

Men's Health
- Best Impotence Health Diet

Weight loss
- Ten (10) Day Quick Success Weight Loss Program: A new approach to losing weight by changing your eating habits for life
- Discover Secret Anti-Aging Juice & Tonic Recipes: Unique Juices And Tonics That Create Beauty And Youth

To see all the kindle books written by this author, go to this the Authors Profile Page or this URL: http://tinyurl.com/b2f7wd3

If you need support or want to promote any of his e-books, please contact him at rss41@yahoo.com and expect a reply within 24 hours. He looks forward to hearing from you and is happy to help you understand his material on natural and nutritional health.

Give A Review

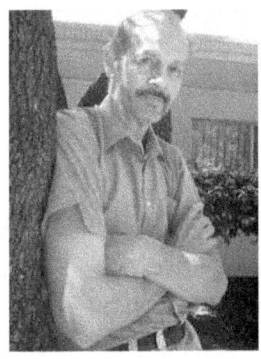

And, don't for get to give a review for this e-book at Amazon so that others can gain the benefits of what is in this e-book. To you, for losing weight, creating better health and more happiness in your life,

Rudy S Silva

www.ingramcontent.com/pod-product-compliance
Lightning Source LLC
Chambersburg PA
CBHW070801290526
45795CB00002B/589